Iodine: The Hidden Chemical at the Center of Your Health and Well-being

Jennifer Cox

presentation of the information is without contract or any type of guarantee assurance.

The trademarks that are used are without any consent, and the publication of the trademark is without permission or backing by the trademark owner. All trademarks and brands within this book are for clarifying purposes only and are the owned by the owners themselves, not affiliated with this document.

DISCLAIMER: This book is for educational and information purposes only. Play it safe and discuss any issues you may have with your physician. Consult your physician before making any diet changes or when using a supplement.

Table of Contents

Introduction – What is Iodine?

If you've ever scraped your knee, or seen a hospital show on television then you've probably seen a brown liquid antiseptic used to clean wounds. This is what most of us associate with iodine. It smells funny, looks weird, and isn't something you've ever probably given a second thought to. Certainly you've never thought of including it in your diet!

Our bodies are composed of a variety of different minerals and chemicals. We know about calcium in our bones, iron in our blood but have you ever heard of iodine being part of that makeup?

In fact, your body needs iodine for several reasons. It's one of the elements that we really don't think about until something goes wrong, yet without it brain development and intellect suffer, and a deficiency can also cause stunted growth, weight issues, and even certain forms of cancer.

The thyroid gland (located just behind your throat) is responsible for all sorts of hormone synthesis and is the primary organ that needs iodine. Iodine helps the thyroid to regulate your metabolism, synthesize necessary hormones, and develop your skeleton and your brain. There's no doubt that iodine is essential to your well-being.

Only a short while ago iodine deficiency was a visible problem, Goiter was a relatively common disease linked to iodine deficiency. Those who suffer from this have a visible swelling around the neck and larynx, all from a simple iodine deficiency. In 1924 the Morton company began adding iodine as a supplement to its salt and so millions were no longer at risk from diseases linked to iodine deficiency.

Iodine is a naturally rare element, found primarily in the ocean. Most people get their daily iodine from supplemented table salt, but less than half of the population are actually getting enough iodine to support their health. The current trend for reducing salt from dietary sources is also cutting iodine out of the equation. Iodine deficiency is an epidemic that no one seems to have heard about.

Despite the obvious health benefits of reduced salt intake, the majority of the population isn't doing anything about losing their only source of iodine. Probably because other than seeing it written on the salt shaker they have absolutely no idea of it's importance.

So, if it's such a big problem but no one has heard of it is it really that big of a deal?

Chapter 1 – The Importance of Minerals

Without proper mineral intake, we would die, and iodine is one of the necessary minerals. So it's a pretty big problem if we're not getting enough of it. Minerals are really that important to the body. Essential minerals are those that fall into this category and they can be divided up into both macrominerals and microminerals.

Each group is important but we need them in different amounts to be healthy. This doesn't necessarily reflect on their importance, they are all important, but without them death and disease are inevitable. A balanced diet usually provides adequate minerals, but even a balanced diet sometimes falls short.

Minerals are as important as vitamins and often the only way you can get most of them is through diet. Many of the minerals we need belong to groups like Halogens. Halogens are normally found in a gaseous state but can be absorbed by the environment so that when we ingest them our bodies can use them as a mineral. The problem is not all minerals work well together, and certain combinations can be detrimental.

Toxic Halogens

Halogens are elements in their own right but are also minerals, though our bodies don't need all the halogens the ones that we do need in our mineral intake can negatively affect the way our bodies process iodine. They are also commonly used in processed foods these days as an alternative to iodine.

Iodine is technically also a halogen but unlike the others, it is actually beneficial. Bromine/bromide has been used in most commercial processes to replace iodine, it's similar chemically but it is actually terribly toxic.

Bromide can exacerbate thyroid issues and will also damage the body's enzyme sodium-iodide-supporter (SIS). It's used in almost all processed foods and even some medications simply because it's cheaper, with the logic that a consumer shouldn't be eating enough of the product to reach toxic levels. Regardless of whether bromide reaches that level, even small amounts are still damaging the thyroid and the body's ability to process iodine.

In the last 30-60 years, many of these halogens have made their way into the food chain. Since they are so chemically close to iodine they're especially dangerous as the body mistakenly accepts them in place of iodine. Think of Halogens as similar sized square blocks, while the square hole is meant for passing iodine blocks through the others will also fit, even if that isn't the purpose.

The hole is then blocked for iodine to use because another block has taken its place. Unlike iodine though these toxic halogens have no way to be excreted from the body and can eventually lead to toxic levels. We don't need these Halogens but we're consuming them anyway and it's damaging our ability to absorb nutrients we do need.

Macrominerals

Macrominerals are Sodium, Chloride, Potassium, Calcium, Phosphorous, Magnesium, and Sulfur. These are all elements that are needed in larger amounts, in comparison, to stave off deficiency diseases. Many of them come from supplemented, processed foods which is why deficiencies are so hard to detect in the western population.

Many macrominerals are found in supplemented cereals and dairy products but just because the packaging says that it has X mineral in it, it doesn't necessarily mean that that mineral is bio-available to the body.

For the body to be able to actually use these minerals they need to be in a type that it can actually use. For example, you might have a pair of jeans but you need blue jeans specifically. Bio-available simply means that the molecule is in a specific form for the body to use.

Many of these minerals are needed for healthy bone structure, nerve transmission, protein synthesis, and muscle health. It's very rare that you'll find people with sodium or chloride deficiencies simply because the western diet is so loaded down with added salt.

Microminerals

Microminerals are often referred to as trace minerals because they are only needed in small amounts. Many of them are metals and if the blood concentration of these becomes too high they can become toxic. The majority of microminerals come from fruits and vegetables. Even though iron is considered to be a trace mineral it's actually needed in sufficient quantity to be considered a macromineral.

Microminerals are Iron, Zinc, Iodine, Selenium, Copper, Manganese, Fluorine, Chromium, and Molybdenum. However, Vanadium, Silicon, Nickel, and Cobalt are also needed in very tiny amounts even though it's not enough to consider them microminerals.

Most microminerals are used for enzyme activity or are antioxidants, iron is the exception because it is needed for red blood cells. Iodine is also unique in that it is wholly used for hormones and development and although these are linked to enzyme activity the mineral itself is not directly used in the formation or workings of enzymes in the body.

Iodine's Importance

As a mineral iodine is responsible for regulating growth, body development, and for metabolism through various hormones and processes. It's usually found in foods grown in iodine-rich soil which explains why so many foods these days are iodine deficient.

 Most commercial growing processes use complex methods like hydroponics to grow food year round without soil, this means that the nutrients of the food only come from whatever fertilizer is added to the water source. Iodine is also found in seafood and some supplemented dairy products.

As with many minerals, deficiency in iodine is linked to a variety of different diseases. Very few people are concerned with their iodine intake because they're more worried about the more well-known minerals like iron. It would be a misconception to believe that iodine is any less important just because it's not as well known.

Chapter 2 – The Functions of Iodine

Iodine is important for the health of the thyroid gland, but the thyroid itself is responsible for a vast amount of systems and regulations across the body. Having an iodine deficiency not only affects the thyroid but many other systems in the body too.

Metabolism/Weight

Iodine is one of the main minerals needed by the thyroid which is ultimately in charge of your metabolism. Your metabolism is used to control how your body burns food/fuel and whether it is used for energy, stored, or used to heat the body.

Without a fully functioning thyroid, this equation can be skewed which is why weight is a common indicator of thyroid health.

Some thyroid diseases like Hashimoto's and Grave's are linked to iodine because of a faulty metabolism. The confirmation of thyroid and metabolism being linked is when people have had their thyroid removed (due to cancer etc.) they are usually told to expect massive weight gain.

Essentially, once the thyroid is removed they have no metabolism of their own and the function must be done using synthetic hormones for the rest of their lives.

Without the thyroid, the body cannot metabolize iodine either since the I^2 molecules need to be split in half before they are bio-available. These molecules are then used to create the hormones needed all over the body by the thyroid gland. Without these hormones, our bodies cannot process food, produce sex hormones, or have proper brain function. The entire body literally depends on the metabolism of iodine into hormones to function.

It's also possible that the Western obesity epidemic may be in part linked to iodine. Iodine's ability to regulate hormones means that it is closely tied to insulin, the hormone regulating blood glucose levels. Since the thyroid hormones and metabolism control weight, not having adequate iodine would be linked to weight gain.

Iodine is mostly stored in fat cells. However, in the fat cells, toxic halogens can replace iodine in the fat cells which makes it difficult to lose the weight. This is because the body doesn't need the halogen molecules, therefore it doesn't break the fat cell down to get to them.

Low thyroid activity can be attributed to modest weight gain. However, without a way to excrete the halogens by breaking down the fat cells boosting thyroid function alone may not help. Saunas and steam rooms are the only way to sweat out these halogens so that the fat has space for bonding with iodine and can be broken down easier.

Mental Development

The World Health Organization has made a strong link between iodine deficiency and a variety of childhood development issues. Mental retardation, developmental delays, and even child mortality are all linked to iodine deficiency.

Iodine works through hormones to develop the nerves and brain tissue. Iodine is used during the nerve insulation process called myelination. This can be especially important during pregnancy and early childhood as seen by the fact that a variety of developmental diseases and birth defects are linked to iodine deficiency. Studies have shown that an iodine deficiency during pregnancy can be linked to a loss of around 10-15 IQ points on average and is considered the largest cause of preventable brain damage.

This is not to say that low iodine is only a problem for pregnant women and babies. In fact, many who suffer from low iodine will talk of a "brain fog". Low iodine causes a rise in the hormone histadine and, therefore, histamine – rather like an allergic reaction.

The histamine causes the brain to struggle by swelling tissues and diverting resources away from major functions for inflammation and other allergic processes. Some foods are naturally high in histadine while others will promote the body to produce it, dairy for example. However, it's most often increased iodine that can quickly remedy this problem.

Fertility

We've seen how iodine can affect fetal development but it's also important even before conception. If the thyroid isn't able to do even the most basic functions because of low iodine it has to work harder. For example, if a woman's estrogen level is too low she may stop ovulating or experience amenorrhea (loss of menstruation) causing infertility.

High blood pressure during pregnancy has also been linked to low iodine levels. Male fertility may also be damaged by low iodine because of the importance of hormones regulated by the thyroid during sperm production.

The main concern of iodine deficiency when it comes to fertility is actually after conception. During pregnancy and birth, a woman needs far more iodine than normal or they risk the child having drastic birth defects.

Immune Function

Iodine plays a role in immune function. As an element, it has known antibacterial, antiviral, anti-parasitic and anticancer properties. Remember when we started? The orange solution spread on wounds? Iodine. High doses of iodine are actually used in radiation therapy to treat breast and thyroid cancer.

Iodine deficiency has also been linked to cysts and infections showing that it could play a role in how efficient the body's response is to pathogens. Much of the immune system is based on glandular responses and inflammation. Without a properly functioning thyroid, this response may never happen. Iodine can also act as a carrier for cells that target and destroy bacteria to reach infected areas.

Chapter 3 – Iodine Deficiency and the Thyroid

Iodine deficiency is linked to many diseases but most of them stem from the fact that iodine is paramount to thyroid health. It is a critical ingredient in the thyroid's production of many hormones.

Iodine has gradually been phased out from the food chain and replaced by cheaper alternatives that are not necessarily better for anyone but profits. While the rate of iodine intake has decreased the amount of thyroid related illnesses and developmental issues has increased dramatically.

For example, while iodine used to be used in commercial bread processes it has been replaced by the cheaper bromine. Instead of adding a nutrient that is necessary, manufacturers are opting for profits and using a gas that is used to fumigate houses instead!

Signs of deficiency

Until we're actually ill, many of us don't notice the small symptoms of mineral deficiency. As parents we worry constantly over every little detail of our children's lives but when it comes to our own any but the most major symptoms are ignored.

Iodine deficiency can be seen in both physical and mental signs though most of them are dismissed as just side effects of our busy lives. For example, lethargy, weight gain, poor memory, headaches, and fatigue are all just another day for most people.

Infertility, early menopause, and menstrual issues are

only a concern of women. Cold hands and an intolerance to cold might be dismissed as simply a sign of the winter season. Until it comes to serious diseases linked to an iodine deficiency most people will simply never notice these early signs.

As we saw earlier, thyroid health is strongly linked to metabolism and weight, weight loss or gain is a significant indicator of your thyroid health. That is not to say that every overweight person has a thyroid issue, but because the hormones produced by the thyroid are part of the metabolic process it can be a strong indicator.

Asides from major metabolic diseases, iodine is also important to the pancreas, adrenal glands, pituitary, and genitals when it comes to hormone production. This could be why there is a link between fertility issues and iodine deficiency.

As well as brittle nails thyroid issues can also manifest as signs on the skin, but again they can be so minute that they are easily dismissed.

Keloids (a type of scarring), hemorrhoids, dry skin and dry hair that falls out frequently are all signs of mineral deficiency linked to iodine. Hair loss is also a strong symptom of iodine deficiency since the thyroid is responsible for growth hormones needed for healthy hair growth.

Iodine deficiency can lead to hair weakness and even hair loss. In 2001 studies were done where patients with alopecia were treated with iodine and in some cases, it was found that patients managed to regrow hair just with supplementation.

Deficiency in Children

Unlike adults, children are often scrutinized at a level where iodine deficiency can be caught early, but their diet is also more likely to be richer in iodine because of supplementation.

Until children are old enough to voice their issues though many more serious diseases are only noticed by doctors when they become a problem. For example, developmental delays and mental retardation are both signs of iodine deficiency.

Down's syndrome has also been linked to iodine deficiency during pregnancy. ADD, PDD, and LD are all linked to thyroid problems and iodine deficiency yet many parents will blame "chemicals" or vaccines for their child's problems.

Conditions Linked to Iodine

Hyperthyroidism and hypothyroidism are both linked to weight and the thyroid gland but only hypothyroidism is connected to Iodine.

Breast cancer, ovarian cancer, and fibrocystic breast disease have also been linked to low iodine because of the thyroid's responsibility to produce necessary hormones in the adrenals and gonads.

Some autoimmune diseases are also linked to poor thyroid function; Grave's and Hashimoto's are both linked to iodine deficiencies by way of the thyroid gland. Even though it is less commonly seen today, goiters are the most obvious sign of iodine deficiency.

Hypothyroidism

Goiter is one of the first indications of hypothyroidism, a condition where the thyroid is simply inadequately able to work with the body's needs.

Hypothyroidism actually affects far more women than men by a rate of about 9 to 1. The reason for this is rather ironic, even though the thyroid is responsible for female hormones it's actually the female hormone estrogen that prevents the body from being able to properly absorb iodine.

Hypothyroidism can also lead to other diseases like cretinism, a disease of stunted growth, mental retardation, and deafness which is usually a birth defect from iodine deficiency.

Perchlorate

Although our bodies need the macromineral chlorine a similar mineral called perchlorate, only one atom away, is actually toxic. It's found in both processed food and naturally in the environment though this is most often because of industrial contamination.

Perchlorate can replace the chlorine we need similar to what bromine does for iodine. For example, the Colorado River, a water source for many, is heavily contaminated with perchlorate.

Public drinking water is often laced with perchlorate and it can even pass on through breast milk to children. It is actually a known cause of hypothyroidism because it displaces iodide in the body's receptors and then damages them so they can't transport iodine anymore.

Added fluorine in tap water has also been linked to iodine displacement and diminished thyroid activity yet it is still a common additive. It has been linked to all the same diseases caused by iodine deficiency.

Ways to Improve Thyroid Function

With all of these potential ways to damage your thyroid, it's important to also understand that protecting your thyroid so that it can adequately process iodine is also important.

Cigarettes contain a toxin known as thiocyanate which has been linked to triggering thyroid disease in those with certain genetic markers. It has also been linked to a tendency for Grave's syndrome and worsening of thyroid activity.

Much of thyroid health is determined by diet so a healthy diet is important to support a working thyroid. A healthy lifestyle that includes exercise may also improve thyroid activity by improved blood flow.

Chapter 4 – Iodine Supplements

It's pretty clear that an iodine deficiency can have dramatic effects on your health. Yet it also seems that getting the recommended amount seems nigh on impossible with the way manufacturers are removing added iodine from food.

It's understandable why many would first turn towards supplementation before trying to fix their diet. After all, this is the easy way since many common multivitamins have iodine in them. In fact, many people have made a rather long leap that taking iodine supplements will help you lose weight by boosting thyroid activity. Despite iodine being a necessity it is still possible to take too much of it.

How much does the body really need?

The RDA of iodine is 150micrograms/150μg, which is actually pretty tiny. This amount increases during pregnancy and doubles during breastfeeding. It's very important to note that this amount is micrograms, *not* milligrams, many supplements actually provide iodine in milligram amounts, far above the recommended dose.

However, the RDA which was set during the 1970's was only intended as a preventative level to protect from goiter and not as an amount to aim for. The level also doesn't take into account the fact that our modern lives mean we are at risk of far greater exposure to toxic halogens that will take the place of iodine in our bodies. The actual amount of iodine you need per day may be slightly higher than someone from 1970.

In fact, during the 1970's it was estimated that from bakery products alone the average intake was 726mcg/day, yet there wasn't a huge prevalence of thyroid issues that the above study would predict. Why?

Not all studies are the same, but if you take the information from the study below and combine it with other studies you'll still see that the recommended amount is far below any that is considered harmful.

The average intake in the Japanese population (mostly from a high seaweed and sea vegetable intake) is about 13.8mg a day, almost a hundred times the American RDA, yet their rates of cancers related to iodine deficiency are far lower.

It's actually estimated that with your iodine intake your body will still excrete up to 90% of it without using it. This means that even though the RDA is low and taking too much might be harmful your body won't store it like Bromine and other harmful halogens.

Too much iodine?

We've established that it's possible to have both an iodine-rich diet and take iodine supplements, too little iodine is obviously harmful but what about too much?

A study in 2011 had participants taking 12 different supplemented doses of iodine from 0-2000mcg/day over the course of 4 weeks. Those participants whose dose was above 400mcg were at greater risk for developing hypothyroidism as the thyroid became overwhelmed.

At 2000mcg participants had a 47% chance of developing hypothyroidism and experienced obvious symptoms. Many daily iodine supplements have 7 times this amount in!

Excess iodine can be harmful, it's unlikely that you'll be allergic to an iodine supplement but hives and anaphylaxis are potential risks if you are.

Toxic iodine levels are usually similar to those from iodine deficiency so it's important to have your levels tested before adding supplementation to make sure you know your numbers. Potentially the response could be from bromine and not iodine in your intake. Acne, fever, headaches, nausea, diarrhea and a rash are all indications of iodine toxicity.

Choosing Iodine Supplements

As noted you're quite likely to see an iodine supplement that has far too much iodine in it. The first thing you'll need to establish is whether you really need supplementation.

If you're not on a low-sodium diet and are taking a multivitamin, then there is only a very small chance that you need an iodine supplement on top of these. Check your multivitamin, chances are there is close to the RDA in it already so you're covered.

If you're looking for an iodine only supplement look for one that is as close to the RDA as you can get, most of the pill will be placebo and filler so choose a reputable brand. Lugol and Ioderol, for example, are thousands of times higher than the upper limit recommended for iodine per day.

Choose a potassium iodide version since this is a much more stable form of the mineral and will give your thyroid some protection from damage as well as a much lower dose.

There is some research that shows a therapeutic dose of up to 12.5mg/day may work for the first month to boost your iodine levels back to normal, but it should be dropped down at the sign of any side effects and for no longer than a month. After a month a maintenance dose of <1mg/day may still be beneficial if you're struggling with maintaining sufficient iodine levels.

Selenium

In 2003, researchers found that selenium had a strong connection to thyroid tissue and its health. If you're taking an iodine supplement it's also a good idea to add a selenium supplement to protect against thyroid diseases such as goiter and Hashimoto's.

Selenium is part of the process the thyroid uses for hormone synthesis but it has also been linked to having a protective role when it comes to overexposure to iodine. In fact, even patients that have normal levels of selenium but suffer from thyroid conditions may see improvement in thyroid function by adding a selenium supplement.

Health Benefits of Supplementation

If you've been tested and found you don't need an iodine supplement don't take one. It will not help your metabolism and may potentially damage your thyroid.

Most of the time you will only need high dose iodine in the event of a nuclear disaster. The FDA's suggested supplementation level, in this case, is only 165mg though this is undoubtedly far too low. Iodine in it's purest form is technically radioactive which is why it can cause such obvious damage to the body in high forms, essentially iodine overdose is radiation poisoning!

While iodine is obviously necessary several other vitamins and minerals can make a difference with your body's ability to absorb it. Fluoride, Chloride, Bromide and other halogens should be avoided as much as possible – check your food labels and tap water for them especially.

Try and optimize your diet and gut flora to eliminate as much of the toxins and free radicals that can impair iodine uptake.

Chapter 5 – Amp up Your Iodine

We've established that over the years iodine supplemented foods are becoming more scarce. If you're eating a low-salt diet and your other foods are no longer supplemented how are you supposed to get enough?

Supplementation may provide the help that most people need but if you'd rather improve your diet than take a pill here's a few options that might help.

From the Sea

The most effective form of bio-available iodine comes from the sea. While sea salt is a common additive for food, the fact that many cut it out from their diet isn't helping.

The ocean has the largest repository of iodine found anywhere and it is especially found in sea plants. Seaweed like kelp and bladderwrack are both able to store very high concentrations of bio-available iodine in their cells.

There is some link that the reason for this may be to protect themselves from the oxidative stress, caused by toxic free-radicals, in our polluted oceans. These seaweeds are ideal for consumption and can be eaten in a variety of different foods. Kelp is available in a noodle/pasta form as well as dried flakes, you can also get it fresh from some supermarkets.

If you are even still using a small amount of salt consider using iodized salt rather than kosher or sea salt as it does still provide some supplementation. Salt will lose 62.4% of its iodine content during the cooking process so consider simply using a little on a salad or raw foods.

Seafood like shrimp, haddock, cod and seabass are all rich in iodine as well. The form of iodine in whole foods like this is much more available than that found in supplemented salt. If you can't make yourself eat seaweed then consider adding fish to your diet 2-3 days a week instead. Sushi and Sashimi are obviously great sources of iodine since you get both fish and seaweed in one!

Grass-Fed Meat & Dairy

Unless they are grown in iodine-rich soil, most plant-based foods have a lower iodine content than animal products. Choosing grass-fed means you're also cutting out free-radicals and other chemicals that might have been introduced to the meat. Organic is suggested for the same reason but if you can't get that just grass-fed will do.

If you're replacing the meat in your diet with soy choose a type that is fermented. The reason for this is that isoflavones found in unfermented soy can impair your thyroid. These antioxidants are more like free-radicals when in your body and are not like the flaviones you'll find in tea.

Most soy-milk products are unfermented, while many block soy products are still safe. For those trying to avoid the problems of dairy, soy can be just as bad. Many soy products are also GMO which means that we're still not sure exactly what they do to your body in the long term.

Avoiding Sources of Bromine/Bromide

Bromide replaces iodine in your body but doesn't do it any good. Many foods are puffed up using bromine as a cheaper alternative. For example, Brominated Vegetable Oil (BVO) is often found in citrus flavored drinks as an additive, not only that but it's also used as a flame retardant! Yuk! Potassium Bromate is also found in many commercial bread products as a dough conditioner as well as many bleached and treated flours.

Try to drink filtered water rather than soda as this will limit your exposure to BVO in drinks and fluoride in tap water. You can simply avoid commercial bread by making your own, it's really easy!

Many commercial chemicals are also responsible for being a source of bromine in your life. Plastic bottles and Tupperware often leach chemicals into the food within. Hair products and cosmetics are especially full of the stuff – dyes, deodorants, even your new clothes might be saturated in them! Remember that even if you don't think you're ingesting it you might be putting it directly on your skin and it's still being absorbed.

Avoiding Hypothyroidism

While it's easier to prevent than treat, hypothyroidism is simply a matter of keeping your thyroid healthy. Avoiding bromine and eating an iodine-rich diet will do a lot towards making sure your thyroid remains healthy.

Staying away from sources of radioactive iodine are also important. Certain foods can also impair thyroid function so they should be eaten in moderation. Broccoli, strawberries, spinach, rutabaga, kale, peaches, cauliflower and peanuts are all goitrogens which can interfere with the thyroid.

Ironically many of these foods also contain high levels of the antioxidant glutathione which has been linked to improvements in those suffering from Hashimoto's disease. It has been linked to actually healing thyroid tissue despite being a goitrogen.

Chapter 6 – Iodine and Health Complications

We've seen that iodine is involved in keeping many systems healthy in the body, but it's also responsible for preventing a variety of diseases too. Without Iodine, we risk cancer and disease in several of the main areas where our bodies should have large stores of this mineral.

Before starting an iodine regiment, it's important to know your levels so that you don't risk overloading your body and damaging the same systems through elevated levels.

Iodine Testing

Iodine testing has to be done through a healthcare provider, there is no "at home" version" but if you're seeing symptoms of iodine deficiency it's certainly something you should consider.

There are three ways to test for iodine and your physician can decide which is best. The most common are blood or urine analysis where a lab will look to detect your iodine levels. This is called a loading test where you'll ingest a specific amount of iodine and then your fluids will be monitored to see how much you excrete. A healthy iodine level is retaining 10% while excreting 90% yet most will see a retention of over 50% and excretion around 40% - a sign of severe deficiency.

Another option is to get a prescription for SSKI (super-saturated potassium iodine). If you rub a few drops of the SSKI solution anywhere on your skin once a day, then touch a wet surface with your fingertips you'll see a yellowish stain left behind if your iodine levels are high.

The reason for this is that your body is saturated and is trying to rid itself of the excess iodine through your pores. It doesn't give you an exact per ml measurement of your iodine levels but if you're getting noticeable staining then you don't need a supplement.

Breast Health

Iodine deficiency has also been linked to a variety of different reproductive issues.

Since breast tissue actually contains a higher level of the body's stored iodine than the thyroid gland it's understandable that iodine issues may be seen in the same tissue. Breasts are made up of proteins that help the thyroid transport iodine through the blood.

Since newborns require higher levels of iodine it makes sense that the method by which a baby feeds is also saturated with iodine. Studies have shown that iodine has an antioxidant effect similar to vitamin C and that without adequate iodine breast tissue begins to show free radical damage that is a factor in breast cancer development.

Problems with iodine in breast tissue can also be linked to cortisol levels as iodine is used to regulate this hormone which has also been linked to impaired immune function. Studies that have compared Western and Japanese diets against the incidence of breast cancer support this. Japanese women have an average iodine intake that is 25 times higher than

Western women and their incidence of breast cancer is also 1/3 lower.

Cardiovascular Health

Even though there is not a direct therapeutic link between iodine intake and heart disease those who eat a diet rich in iodine tend to have a lower risk for hypertension and heart disease.

The thyroid controls lipid profiles through hormones and enzymes and without proper regulation these can become imbalanced. Hypothyroidism has been linked to a higher risk for stroke and heart disease. LDL and atherosclerosis are both increased with poor thyroid function, this can also weaken the heart muscle and cause cardiac arrhythmia.

Therapies using iodine have shown improvement in patients and a lowering of risk factors for cardiovascular disease.

Cancer Preventative?

With iodine having antioxidant properties it's quite possible that it can be linked to preventing a variety of different cancers.

Many of the tissues that should be saturated in iodine become damaged when deficient which raises the risk of certain cancers. Breast, Thyroid, Prostate and Stomach cancer are all linked to iodine deficiencies. Stomach lining cells, for example, are particularly rich in iodine and research has made some tenuous links between digestive cancers and iodine deficiency.

Those who are iodine deficient are not only at risk for

goiters but also have a much higher risk for stomach cancer. There is a strong conclusion with this research that the two are directly related.

Harmful Iodine

Not all sources of iodine are good. Iodine in it's purest form is radioactive and this is used by the medical industry for a variety of therapies.

Nuclear power plant contamination is also largely made of radioactive iodine. Organic iodine can be harmful but it is less likely to cause the same issues. Radioactive iodine is linked to thyroid cancers and even some other rare cancers.

If you're worried about your radiation exposure (due to living in a location near a plant, or on a granite neighborhood, then consider getting a Geiger meter and testing the levels for your own safety.

If you are getting X-rays for surgical reasons ask for a Thyroid collar, if possible, to help protect your thyroid from any radiation. Most technicians will not use or offer these unless you ask but without one, you're needlessly exposing your thyroid to radiation that is potentially damaging.

Chapter 7 – Iodine Induced Hyperthyroidism

Just as having too little iodine can be bad for you so too can excess iodine. Too much iodine can damage the thyroid and cause hypothyroidism but it can also cause hyperthroidism as well.

The difference is that in hyperthyroidism the thyroid goes into overdrive and produces too many hormones. In this case, it can be too much of a good thing and the body is just as damaged. The phenomena is known as the Jod-Basedow Phenomenon and it is common in locations where people are iodine deficient.

Ironically it seems you can have both extremes from one deficiency. It has also been diagnosed frequently in travelers who use iodine enriched water or purification supplements as well as overuse of topical iodine for antibacterial purposes.

One of the biggest problems of iodine-induced hyperthyroidism is that those who mistakenly believe they suffer from an iodine deficiency begin to self-medicate using supplements that are too high. This can confuse the thyroid and overload it meaning it loses the ability to regulate exactly how much hormones are required by the body.

Iodine Overload

We've seen that too much iodine can be just as problematic as a deficiency. Overloading the body with iodine means that it will start to be excreted from your pores but it can also have drastic effects on your thyroid process too. When your iodine levels are too high your thyroid may no longer be sensitive to the hormone thyroxine that regulates it to process the iodine. Thyroxine hormone is produced and regulated by the thyroid, so it is essential for the health of your thyroid.

The process similar to how type 2 diabetes works with insulin hormone sensitivity. The process may only last for several days at a time which is why it's so hard to diagnose. The thyroid may then start to release a rush of hormones to counter it.

Without proper regulation however, the thyroid is not able to continue to produce hormones when needed and will often continue to pump out high levels of thyroxine. There is, however, a chance that the thyroid is still functioning normally but the lack of thyroxine control is because of damaged tissue acting autonomously.

Autonomous Nodules

Another cause of hyperthyroidism is the development of autonomous thyroid nodules – thyroid tissue that works independently from the thyroid itself.

While the hormone thyroxine, released into the blood stream, will staunch thyroid activity once iodine uptake is sufficient any autonomous nodule will remain unaffected.

Thyroid function might be sufficient and even indicative of low-iodine. These nodules are mutated, cloned cells from the thyroid. They are usually cloned from Thyroid Stimulating Hormone Receptor cells becoming damaged by iodine deficiency and then multiplying uncontrollably.

Without proper diagnosis iodine uptake is unregulated and can skyrocket to levels of toxicity even if thyroid activity is deemed normal. The only solution for this is to deactivate or remove the nodule.

These nodules are actually relatively rare and it's thought that those who do manifest hyperthyroidism may have already been suffering from damaged thyroid function due to iodine deficiency.

Conclusion

Iodine is an essential mineral that the body needs to stay healthy. Whether it is found in raised amounts or deficient, iodine can have a huge effect on thyroid health. It is most plentiful in the sea which is why many land grown foods are deficient in iodine.

It is used by the thyroid to moderate and manufacture hormones but is also found in concentration in breast tissue. Even though it's primary use is for hormonal balance, iodine is also used for many reproductive processes.

Iodine is only found in few foodstuffs and with many modern processes swapping iodine for bromine, a large portion of the population are losing out on this important nutrient. Even though so many in the population are deficient, few people really know anything about their iodine levels or what this mineral does.

Iodine has been linked to many thyroid related diseases. These can mean overactive and underactive thyroid activity, and they are equally dangerous. Thyroid issues are especially dangerous for women who are pregnant or nursing as the result can be severe birth defects and even life-shortening to the child. Even a small iodine deficiency at this time can cause a moderate drop in IQ.

Hypo and Hyperthyroidism are both common problems from iodine levels. They are often diagnosed by massive shifts in weight level and need to be controlled by daily hormones or even surgery in extreme cases. Nodules can also form on the thyroid which act independently causing these conditions even though thyroid activity remains normal.

Levels of iodine have also been linked to a variety of different cancers. Whether iodine supplements can act as a preventative has not been determined yet but many supplements are not sufficient to solve the average iodine deficiency.

It's very possible to have too much of a good thing with iodine and as a micromineral, the body really doesn't need a lot in a supplement. Many supplements have hundreds of times the necessary amount of iodine in them so it's important when picking a supplement that you check the dosage. When taking an iodine supplement it's also a good idea to add selenium or another brain function mineral supplement like DHA.

It's quite clear that without iodine we would die, but even if we're scraping by on the RDA we're still not doing our bodies any good.

Consider getting your iodine levels checked so you can make an informed choice about how much iodine you need, especially if you're considering pregnancy.

Iodine might not be the most well-known mineral but it's just as important!